THE COMPLETE GUIDE TO HERBAL SUPPLEMENTS

Understanding the Science Behind Natural Health

Peirce Maureen

INTRODUCTION

CHAPTER ONE

THE SCIENCE OF HERBAL MEDICINE

CHAPTER TWO

POPULAR HERBAL SUPPLEMENTS

CHAPTER THREE

CHOOSING QUALITY HERBAL SUPPLEMENTS

CHAPTER FOUR

THE REGULATORY LANDSCAPE

CHAPTER FIVE

HERBAL SUPPLEMENTS AND DRUG INTERACTIONS

CHAPTER SIX

HERBAL SUPPLEMENTS AND SPECIFIC HEALTH CONDITIONS

CHAPTER SEVEN

INCORPORATING HERBAL SUPPLEMENTS INTO YOUR WELLNESS PLAN

CHAPTER EIGHT

CONCLUSION

INTRODUCTION

The introduction to "The Complete Guide to Herbal Supplements: Understanding the Science Behind Natural Health" is a critical chapter that provides a foundation for the rest of the book. It covers essential information about herbal supplements, including their history, benefits, and safety considerations.

The chapter begins with an overview of the use of herbal remedies throughout history, from ancient civilizations to modern times. Readers will learn how herbal medicine has been used to treat various health conditions and promote overall wellness for thousands of years.

The chapter also explores the potential benefits of herbal supplements, including their ability to support overall health and wellness, boost the immune system, and improve specific health conditions. Readers will learn about the various types of herbal supplements available and how they work to support the body's natural functions.

Safety considerations are also discussed in this chapter. While herbal supplements are generally considered safe, there are potential risks associated with their use. Readers will learn about the importance of consulting with a healthcare provider before using herbal supplements, potential side effects, and risks associated with certain herbs.

Overall, the Introduction to Herbal Supplements provides a broad overview of the history and benefits of herbal medicine, while also emphasizing the importance of safety and caution when using herbal supplements. It sets the stage for the rest of the book, which delves deeper into the science behind herbal medicine and provides practical guidance for safe and effective use of herbal supplements.

CHAPTER ONE

The Science of Herbal Medicine

"The Science of Herbal Medicine" is a critical chapter in "The Complete Guide to Herbal Supplements: Understanding the Science Behind Natural Health." In this chapter, readers will learn about the scientific principles behind herbal medicine and how herbs interact with the body.

The chapter begins by discussing the active ingredients in herbs, which are responsible for their therapeutic effects. These active ingredients are often complex molecules that can be challenging to isolate and study. However, modern scientific techniques have allowed researchers to identify and study these compounds, leading to a better understanding of how they work.

The chapter then explores how herbs interact with the body, including the various ways they can be absorbed, metabolized, and eliminated. Readers will learn about the different mechanisms by which herbs can affect the body, including through their effects on specific cells, organs, and systems.

The chapter also covers the role of traditional knowledge in herbal medicine, including the use of plants by indigenous cultures for medicinal purposes. Readers will learn about the importance of preserving this traditional knowledge while also incorporating modern scientific techniques to better understand the therapeutic effects of herbs.

Overall, "The Science of Herbal Medicine" provides readers with a foundational understanding of the scientific principles behind herbal medicine. By understanding how herbs interact with the body, readers can make more informed decisions about the use of herbal supplements and better understand the potential risks and benefits. This chapter sets the stage for the rest of the book, which explores the specific herbs and their potential uses for various health conditions.

CHAPTER TWO

Popular Herbal Supplements

"Popular Herbal Supplements" is a critical chapter in "The Complete Guide to Herbal Supplements: Understanding the Science Behind Natural Health." In this chapter, readers will learn about some of the most popular herbal supplements, including their potential health benefits and recommended uses.

The chapter covers several widely used herbs, including echinacea, ginseng, St. John's Wort, valerian root, and turmeric. For each herb, readers will learn about its history, traditional uses, and the specific active ingredients that are responsible for its therapeutic effects.

Echinacea is a popular herb often used to boost the immune system and help fight off colds and other respiratory infections. The chapter covers its potential benefits, including reducing the duration and severity of colds, and its active ingredients that help support the immune system.

Ginseng is another popular herb, known for its ability to reduce stress, increase energy, and support mental function. The chapter explores the different types of ginseng, their active ingredients, and how they can help improve cognitive function, reduce fatigue, and promote overall well-being.

St. John's Wort is an herb commonly used to treat mild to moderate depression, anxiety, and sleep disorders. Readers will learn about its active ingredients, including hypericin, and how they help regulate neurotransmitter activity in the brain, leading to improved mood and decreased anxiety.

Valerian root is often used to promote relaxation and treat anxiety and sleep disorders. The chapter covers its potential benefits, including reducing the time it takes to fall asleep and improving the quality of sleep, and its active ingredients, which help regulate the activity of the neurotransmitter GABA.

Turmeric is a potent anti-inflammatory herb often used to treat joint pain and improve overall joint health. Readers will learn about its active ingredient, curcumin, and how it helps reduce inflammation and oxidative stress, leading to improved joint health and reduced pain.

Overall, the chapter on "Popular Herbal Supplements" provides readers with a comprehensive overview of some of the most widely used herbs and their potential health benefits. By understanding the specific uses and active ingredients of these herbs, readers can make more informed decisions about the use of herbal supplements and better understand their potential risks and benefits.

CHAPTER THREE

Choosing Quality Herbal Supplements

"Choosing Quality Herbal Supplements" is a crucial chapter in "The Complete Guide to Herbal Supplements: Understanding the Science Behind Natural Health." In this chapter, readers will learn how to identify high-quality herbal supplements and avoid potentially harmful or ineffective products.

The chapter begins by discussing the importance of sourcing and manufacturing processes in producing high-quality herbal supplements. Readers will learn about the different types of manufacturing processes used to create herbal supplements, including extraction methods and quality control measures. The chapter also covers the importance of third-party testing and certification in ensuring the quality and safety of herbal supplements.

The chapter also explores the different forms in which herbal supplements are available, including capsules, tablets, tinctures, and teas. Readers will learn about the pros and cons of each form, as well as the specific factors that can affect the quality and effectiveness of different forms of herbal supplements.

Readers will also learn about the specific factors to consider when choosing a herbal supplement, including the reputation of the manufacturer, the type and quality of the ingredients used, and the product's labeling and packaging. The chapter covers important details to look for on supplement labels, such as the amount of the active ingredient per serving and the standardization of the herb.

Finally, the chapter provides readers with tips for safely using herbal supplements, including information on dosages, potential side effects, and interactions with prescription medications. Readers will also learn about the importance of consulting with a healthcare professional before using herbal supplements, particularly if they have a pre-existing medical condition or are taking medications.

Overall, "Choosing Quality Herbal Supplements" provides readers with the information they need to make informed decisions about the quality and safety of herbal supplements. By understanding the factors that affect the quality and effectiveness of herbal supplements, readers can choose products that are safe, effective, and appropriate for their individual needs.

CHAPTER FOUR

The Regulatory Landscape

"The Regulatory Landscape" is an important chapter in "The Complete Guide to Herbal Supplements: Understanding the Science Behind Natural Health." In this chapter, readers will learn about the regulatory framework governing the production, marketing, and labeling of herbal supplements.

The chapter begins by providing an overview of the various agencies responsible for regulating the herbal supplement industry, including the Food and Drug Administration (FDA), the Federal Trade Commission (FTC), and the United States Department of Agriculture (USDA). Readers will learn about the specific roles of each agency in ensuring the safety and quality of herbal supplements.

The chapter also covers the regulations governing the labeling of herbal supplements. Readers will learn about the information that must be included on supplement labels, such as the name of the supplement, the amount of active ingredient per serving, and any warnings or contraindications. The chapter also explores the use of health claims and other marketing language on supplement labels, including the requirements for substantiating such claims.

Readers will also learn about the Good Manufacturing Practices (GMPs) established by the FDA to ensure the quality and safety of herbal supplements. The chapter covers the specific requirements of GMPs, including the establishment of written procedures for manufacturing, packaging, and labeling, and the use of quality control measures throughout the production process.

Finally, the chapter explores the potential risks associated with herbal supplements, including contamination, adulteration, and interactions with prescription medications. Readers will learn about the importance of reporting adverse events associated with the use of herbal supplements to the FDA, and how to identify and report potential safety concerns.

Overall, "The Regulatory Landscape" provides readers with an understanding of the complex and evolving regulatory environment governing the herbal supplement industry. By understanding the specific regulations and requirements governing the production, marketing, and labeling of herbal supplements, readers can make more informed decisions about the safety and effectiveness of the supplements they choose to use.

CHAPTER FIVE

Herbal Supplements and Drug Interactions

"Herbal Supplements and Drug Interactions" is a critical chapter in "The Complete Guide to Herbal Supplements: Understanding the Science Behind Natural Health." In this chapter, readers will learn about the potential interactions between herbal supplements and prescription medications.

The chapter begins by providing an overview of the various types of drug interactions that can occur between herbal supplements and prescription medications, including pharmacokinetic and pharmacodynamic interactions. Readers will learn about the factors that can affect the absorption, distribution, metabolism, and elimination of both herbal supplements and prescription medications, and how these factors can lead to potential interactions.

The chapter also covers specific examples of herbal supplements that are known to interact with prescription medications, including St. John's wort, echinacea, and ginkgo biloba. Readers will learn about the specific prescription medications that can be affected by these supplements, as well as the potential risks and side effects of such interactions.

Readers will also learn about the importance of consulting with a healthcare professional before using herbal supplements, particularly if they are taking prescription medications. The chapter covers important considerations for healthcare professionals, including the need to review a patient's medication history and potential risks of interactions before recommending herbal supplements.

Finally, the chapter provides readers with tips for safely using herbal supplements in conjunction with prescription medications, including information on dosages, timing of administration, and potential side effects. Readers will also learn about the importance of monitoring for any potential changes in symptoms or medication effects when using herbal supplements.

Overall, "Herbal Supplements and Drug Interactions" provides readers with the information they need to make informed decisions about the safe use of herbal supplements in conjunction with prescription medications. By understanding the potential risks and interactions associated with using herbal supplements, readers can work with their healthcare professionals to ensure safe and effective use of both prescription medications and herbal supplements.

CHAPTER SIX

Herbal Supplements and Specific Health Conditions

"Herbal Supplements and Specific Health Conditions" is an important chapter in "The Complete Guide to Herbal Supplements: Understanding the Science Behind Natural Health." In this chapter, readers will learn about the potential benefits and risks of using herbal supplements to support specific health conditions.

The chapter begins by providing an overview of the specific health conditions that may benefit from the use of herbal supplements. This includes conditions such as anxiety, depression, arthritis, and digestive disorders, among others. Readers will learn about the specific herbs and supplements that may be beneficial for each condition, as well as the potential risks and side effects of such supplements.

The chapter covers some of the most commonly used herbal supplements for specific health conditions, including chamomile for anxiety and sleep disorders, St. John's wort for depression, and ginger for nausea and vomiting. Readers will learn about the potential benefits of these supplements, as well as the potential risks and side effects associated with their use.

Readers will also learn about the importance of consulting with a healthcare professional before using herbal supplements to support specific health conditions. The chapter covers important considerations for healthcare professionals, including the need to review a patient's medical history, potential drug interactions, and potential risks of interactions with prescription medications.

Finally, the chapter provides readers with tips for safely using herbal supplements to support specific health conditions, including information on dosages, timing of administration, and potential side effects. Readers will also learn about the importance of monitoring for any potential changes in symptoms or medication effects when using herbal supplements to support specific health conditions.

Overall, "Herbal Supplements and Specific Health Conditions" provides readers with the information they need to make informed decisions about the safe and effective use of herbal supplements to support specific health conditions. By understanding the potential benefits and risks of using herbal supplements for specific health conditions, readers can work with their healthcare professionals to develop a safe and effective treatment plan.

CHAPTER SEVEN

Incorporating Herbal Supplements into Your Wellness Plan

"Incorporating Herbal Supplements into Your Wellness Plan" is an important chapter in "The Complete Guide to Herbal Supplements: Understanding the Science Behind Natural Health." In this chapter, readers will learn about the benefits of using herbal supplements as part of a comprehensive wellness plan.

The chapter begins by providing an overview of the various aspects of wellness that can be supported by herbal supplements. This includes physical wellness, emotional wellness, and spiritual wellness, among others. Readers will learn about the potential benefits of herbal supplements for each of these aspects of wellness, as well as the importance of incorporating them into a comprehensive wellness plan.

The chapter covers some of the most commonly used herbal supplements for overall wellness, including ginseng, turmeric, and ashwagandha. Readers will learn about the potential benefits of these supplements, as well as the potential risks and side effects associated with their use.

Readers will also learn about the importance of developing a personalized wellness plan that incorporates herbal supplements in a safe and effective manner. The chapter provides tips for developing a wellness plan, including setting goals, identifying potential barriers, and creating a comprehensive plan that includes exercise, nutrition, and stress reduction techniques.

Finally, the chapter provides readers with tips for incorporating herbal supplements into their wellness plan, including information on dosages, timing of administration, and potential side effects. Readers will also learn about the importance of monitoring for any potential changes in symptoms or medication effects when using herbal supplements as part of a wellness plan.

Overall, "Incorporating Herbal Supplements into Your Wellness Plan" provides readers with the information they need to make informed decisions about the safe and effective use of herbal supplements as part of a comprehensive wellness plan. By understanding the potential benefits and risks of using herbal supplements for overall wellness, readers can work with their healthcare professionals to develop a personalized plan that supports their overall health and wellbeing.

CHAPTER EIGHT

Conclusion

In conclusion, "The Complete Guide to Herbal Supplements: Understanding the Science Behind Natural Health" is an essential resource for anyone seeking to improve their health and wellbeing through the use of herbal supplements. Through its comprehensive exploration of the science behind herbal medicine, this guide empowers readers to make informed decisions about the safe and effective use of herbal supplements.

With its detailed exploration of the benefits and risks of specific herbal supplements for various health conditions, this guide provides readers with the knowledge they need to work with their healthcare professionals to develop a safe and effective treatment plan. Furthermore, the guide's coverage of topics such as the regulatory landscape and potential drug interactions ensures that readers have a complete understanding of the complexities of herbal medicine.

Whether readers are seeking to support specific health conditions or to incorporate herbal supplements into a comprehensive wellness plan, "The Complete Guide to Herbal Supplements" provides the information they need to do so in a safe and effective manner. By understanding the science behind herbal medicine, readers can make informed decisions about the use of herbal supplements and take control of their own health and wellbeing.

We hope that this guide has been informative and useful in your journey towards improved health and wellbeing. Remember, the safe and effective use of herbal supplements requires knowledge and guidance from a healthcare professional. By working together, we can harness the power of herbal medicine to support our health and vitality.

www.ingramcontent.com/pod-product-compliance
Lightning Source LLC
Chambersburg PA
CBHW061558250726
48657CB00021B/2291